Inter

How To Lose Weight Without Exercise, Boost Energy, Reverse Diabetes

(Plant Based Diet Of Weight Loss For Beginners)

Leon Webster

Table Of Contents

Leon Webster 1

Table Of Contents 2

Introduction 1

Greek Breakfast Wraps 6

Parmesan Fresh Freshfresh Eggs Toast With Tomatoes 8

Curried Chicken Breast Wraps 10

Baked Salmon Fillets With Tomato And Mushrooms 11

Protein Power Sweet Potatoes 13

Avocado And Fennel Salad With Balsamic Vinaigrette 15

Penne Pasta With Vegetables 16

Hearty Shrimp And Kale Soup (26 0 Calories Per Serving) 19

Pork Loin Chops With Mango Salsa 21

Lemon-Sesame Chicken And Asparagus 23

Spinach And 26

Swiss Cheese Omelet 26

Grilled Chicken Salad With Poppy Seed Dressing 28

Quick Miso Soup With Bok Choy And Shrimp. 29

Broiled Halibut With Garlic Spinach 31

Keto Bagel 33

Freshfresh Eggs In The Zucchini Nest 36

Bacon Cauliflower Pan 39

Muffins As Spinach Quiche 40

Pizza Waffles 42

Bacon Freshfresh Eggs In An Avocado Bed ... 44

Mexican Pan 45

Burger With Filling 47

Salmon On Zucchini Pasta 49

Cauliflower Pizza 51

Green Smoothie 54

Spinach Parmesan Bakedfresh Eggs 55

Hummus Breakfast Bowl 57

Mango Smoothie	59
French Toast	59
Burgers, Grass-Fed Style	61
Salmon And Vegetables	62
Fish Tacos	64
Turkey Burrito Skillet	66
Baked Lemon Salmon	68
Broccoli And Chicken Stir Fry	70
Garlic & Honey Shrimp Fry	73
Cod And Moroccan Couscous	75
Chicken Parm Stuffed Peppers	77
Zucchini Enchiladas	79
Avocado Toast	81
Shrimp And Avocado Salad,	82
Breakfast - Italian Melt Omelet	86
Mango Smoothie	88
Steak Taco Bowl	90
Breakfast Burrito	92

Tricolore Salad 94

Dinner - Mexican Tacos 95

Vanilla Smoothie... 97

Spinach Parmesan Bakedfresh Eggs 98

Bacon, Chicken, And Spinach Salad 100

Breakfast - Bacon,Fresh Eggs , And Avocado 102

Bacon Wrapped Chicken Parcels 104

Chorizo, Chicken, And Avocado Salad 106

Breakfast - Chocolate Coconut Smoothie....... 108

Green Smoothie... 110

Dinner - Everything Bowl 112

Breakfast - Caprese Omelet................................. 114

Chicken Salad 116

Dinner - Crispy Thyme & Lemon Chicken 118

Full English Breakfast... 120

Dinner - Italian Melt Omelet 122

Dinner - Chicken And Blackberry Salad 124

Chocolate Smoothie 126

Mediterranean Chicken Risotto 127

Sardine Stuffed Avocado 130

Omelet 132

Black Bean, Cilantro, And Avocado Quesadillas
.... 134

Tuna Quinoa Cakes 136

Slow Cooker Seafood Ramen 138

Slow Grilled Chinese Char Siu Chicken 140

Thai Salad Bowls 142

New Orleans Barbecue Shrimp 145

Creamy Kabocha Squash And Roasted Red
Pepper Pasta 147

Loaded Cauliflower 152

Sweet And Hearty Beef Stew 155

Chocolate Chip Protein Bars 157

Easy Creamy Cajun Shrimp Pasta 160

Gluten-Free Breakfast Skillet 164

Healthy Chicken Taco Soup 167

Citrus Baked Salmon 170

Caribbean Steamed Fish 172

Orange And Green Smoothie 175

Corn Chowder Con Chile Poblano 177

Crispy Potato Tacos 178

Kale And Broccoli Salmon Burgers 181

Grilled Bulgogi Rice Bowls 182

Black Garlic, Sesame, And Shitake Cod 185

Healthy Mexican Casserole 187

Shrimp Lettuce Wraps 191

Shakshuka 194

Coconut Steel-Cut Oatmeal With Almonds And Dark Chocolate 196

Crunchy Roasted Chickpeas 197

Crispy Baked Falafel 198

Introduction

Nowadays the public is overwhelmed by new and innovative diet forms and weight loss programs. As someone who has struggled with the topic himself since his youth, I can say from my own experience that it is mostly about special diets that can lead to the desired success in the short term, but in the long term, no healthy and sustainable change in diet cause.

It was only when I delved deeper into the subject of health a few years ago that I understood how diet can actually have a positive effect on our health, our well-being and our physical fitness.

As a result, I learned to recognize which diets are unhealthy for humans and which can hardly be implemented in the long term. In particular, diets that are based only on individual foods, such as B. the cabbage soup diet are anything but healthy for humans in the long run.

Usually such one-sided diets lead to the deprivation of important micronutrients from the body and deficiency symptoms develop. It is obvious that such a way of life cannot be healthy in the long term.

In the search for a way to achieve your own desired weight and, above all, to keep it permanently, we come across countless forms of nutrition that promise fast, permanent and, last but not least, healthy weight reduction. Reason enough to take a closer look at these forms of nutrition and take a critical look at them. In this guide, we therefore look at what is known as intermittent fasting.

A nutritional concept that has recently gained a lot of attention and is now being increased popularity, especially with athletes (especially in the fitness area).

Even at the risk of the advisor losing some of its tension, I would like to inform you at this point that I consider intermittent fasting among all diets of our day to be a really very useful concept.

In addition to numerous health benefits that intermittent fasting brings, it is also relatively easy to implement and offers a high level of practicality in everyday life.

While just a few years ago the trend was to split our food intake into several small meals over the entire day, intermittent fasting reverses this trend. It is easy to implement, simplifies our everyday life and can help us lose weight permanently in a healthy way.

The low carb diet, a diet in which the amount of carbohydrates consumed is severely restricted, is also becoming increasingly popular in our society.

Both intermittent fasting and the low carb diet have many advantages for us he goal of losing weight and maintaining our desired weight permanently.

In this guide you will find out exactly how this works and how these two forms of nutrition can best be combined.

The first part of the guide deals with intermittent fasting, also called intermittent fasting. What methods are there and why does it make sense to take food breaks at all?

The second part of the guide is dedicated to the classic low carb diet and how this type of diet can help us lose weight successfully. How does low carb work? And how does reducing carbohydrates affect our health?

Together, these two forms of nutrition form the key to a healthy and lean body. That is why I have developed two nutrition plans for you from a combination of intermittent fasting and a low carb diet. These are explained in detail in the third part of this guide.

Greek Breakfast Wraps

This recipe is just as satisfying as that fast-food breakfast sandwich, but this wrap has far less fat and fewer calories. It's a great breakfast to make ahead of time and reheat in the morning or when you get to work.

- 2 teaspoon olive oil

- 1 cup fresh baby spinach leaves • 2 tablespoon fresh basil

- 5 fresh freshfresh eggs whites, beaten

- 1 teaspoon salt

- 1/2 teaspoon freshly ground black pepper

- 1/2 cup crumbed low-fat feta cheese • 2 whole wheat tortillas

1. In a small skillet, heat the olive oil over medium heat. Add the spinach and basil to the pan and sauté for about 2 minutes, or just until the spinach is wilted.
2. Add the fresh freshfresh eggs whites to the pan, season with the salt and pepper, and sauté, stirring often, for about 2 minutes more, or until the egg whites are firm.
3. Remove from the heat and sprinkle with the feta cheese.
4. Heat the tortillas in the microwave for 35 to 40 seconds, or just until softened and warm. Divide the freshfresh eggs between the tortillas and wrap up burrito-style.

Parmesan Fresh Freshfresh Eggs Toast With Tomatoes

This breakfast is quick to make and delicious to eat. You can substitute grape tomatoes if you have them on hand. They provide a healthy dose of vitamin C to your meal.

- 1/2 teaspoon freshly ground black pepper
- 2 large freshfresh eggs
- 2 slices reduced-calorie whole wheat toast
- 2 tablespoon shredded Parmesan cheese
- 2 teaspoon olive oil
- 1 teaspoon chopped garlic (about 2 clove)
- 6 cherry tomatoes, quartered • 1 teaspoon salt

1. In a small skillet, heat the olive oil over medium heat.
2. Add the garlic and tomatoes to the pan and sauté for 2 minutes, stirring often. Season with the salt and pepper, then transfer to a plate to keep warm.
3. In the same skillet, fry the eggs for 2 minutes. Turn over and cook to the desired doneness.
4. Place 2 fresh freshfresh eggs on each slice of toast, top with half the tomatoes, and sprinkle with half the Parmesan cheese.

Curried Chicken Breast Wraps

These quick and filling wraps deliver a lot of flavor for very few calories. Make the filling ahead of time to have on hand for work lunches and busy days.

- 2 small Gala or Granny Smith apple, cored and chopped

- 2 cup spring lettuce mix or baby lettuce

- 2 (8-inch) whole wheat tortillas

- 6 ounces cooked chicken breast, cubed

- 2 tablespoons plain low-fat yogurt • 2 teaspoon Dijon mustard

- 1 teaspoon mild curry powder

In a small bowl, combine the chicken, yogurt, Dijon mustard, and curry powder; stir well to combine. Add the apple and stir until blended.

Divide the lettuce between the tortillas and top each with half of the chicken mixture. Roll up burrito-style and serve.

Yields 2 servings.

Baked Salmon Fillets With Tomato And Mushrooms

Salmon is a great source of healthy fats, especially omega-5 fatty acids. When baked with a mixture of tangy tomatoes and mild mushrooms, it's as delicious as it is healthy.

- 1 teaspoon chopped fresh dill
- 1 cup diced fresh tomato
- 1 cup sliced fresh mushrooms

- 2 (4-ounce) skin-on salmon fillets
- 2 teaspoons olive oil, divided
- 1 teaspoon salt
- 1/2 teaspoon freshly ground black pepper

Preheat the oven to 490 degrees F and line a baking sheet with aluminum foil.

Using your fingers or a pastry brush, coat both sides of the fillets with 1 teaspoon of the olive oil each. Place the salmon skin-side down on the pan. Sprinkle evenly with the salt and pepper.

In a small bowl, combine the remaining 2 teaspoon olive oil, the dill, tomato, and mushrooms; stir well to combine. Spoon the mixture over the fillets.

Fold the sides and ends of the foil up to seal the fish, place the pan on the middle oven rack, and bake for about 25 minutes, or until the salmon flakes easily.

Yields 2 servings.

Protein Power Sweet Potatoes

This recipe is extremely simple and quick, but it packs almost ten grams of protein per serving, which makes it a perfect fasting-day meal for keeping you full and helping you stay energized and focused.

- 2 medium sweet potatoes
- 6 ounces plain Greek yogurt
- 1 teaspoon salt
- 2 /5   cup dried cranberries
- 1/2 teaspoon freshly ground black pepper

Preheat the oven to 400 degrees F and pierce the sweet potatoes several times with a fork. Place them on a baking sheet dish and bake for 40 to 46 minutes, or until easily pierced with a fork.

Cut the potatoes in half and spoon the flesh into a medium mixing bowl, keeping the skins intact. Add the salt, pepper, yogurt, and cranberries to the bowl and mix well with a fork.

Spoon the mixture back into the potato skins and serve warm. Yields 2 servings.

Avocado And Fennel Salad With Balsamic Vinaigrette

This salad is a wonderful blend of tangy citrus, silky avocado, and anise-flavored fennel. Tossed with a quick and easy balsamic vinaigrette, it's a perfect lunch or light supper for warm days.

- 1 avocado, diced
- 1 cup mandarin oranges, drained
- 2 cup chopped romaine lettuce
- 1/2 teaspoon freshly ground black pepper
- 2 tablespoon light olive oil
- 2 tablespoon balsamic vinegar
- 1/2 teaspoon salt
- 1 cup fennel, sliced

In a medium mixing bowl, combine the olive oil, balsamic vinegar, salt, and pepper, and whisk until well combined and slightly thickened. This is your balsamic vinaigrette.

Add the fennel, avocado, oranges, and lettuce; toss until the vegetables are well coated with dressing. Divide between two salad plates and serve cold.

Yields 2 servings.

Penne Pasta With Vegetables

Even on fasting days, you can enjoy a light pasta meal. This one is chock-full of vitamin C and iron from the spinach and tomatoes and delivers lots of flavor and satisfaction.

- 25 cherry tomatoes, halved
- 2 cup fresh spinach leaves
- 1 teaspoon freshly ground black pepper
- 2 tablespoon shredded Parmesan cheese

- 2 teaspoon salt, divided
- 1/3 cup uncooked penne pasta
- 2 tablespoon olive oil
- 2 tablespoon chopped garlic
- 2 teaspoon chopped fresh oregano
- 2 cup sliced fresh mushrooms

In a large saucepan, bring 2 quart water to a boil. Add 1 teaspoon of the salt and the penne, and cook according to package directions, or until al dente (about 10 minutes). Drain but do not rinse the penne, reserving about 1/2 cup pasta water.

Meanwhile, in a large skillet, heat the olive oil over medium-high heat. Add the garlic, oregano, and mushrooms, and sauté for 5 to 6 minutes, or until the mushrooms are golden.

Add the tomatoes and spinach, season with the remaining 1 teaspoon salt and the black pepper, and sauté for 5 to 5 minutes, or until the spinach is wilted.

Add the drained pasta to the skillet, along with 2 to 5 tablespoons of the pasta water. Cook, stirring constantly, for 2 to 5 minutes, or until the pasta is glistening and the water has cooked off.

Divide the pasta between two shallow bowls and sprinkle with the Parmesan cheese. Serve hot or at room temperature.

Hearty Shrimp And Kale Soup
(26 0 Calories Per Serving)

- 8 medium (5 6-40 count) raw shrimp, peeled and halved
- 2 cup canned great northern beans, drained
- 1/2 cup chopped fresh parsley
- 1/2 teaspoon freshly ground black pepper
- 2 teaspoon olive oil
- 2 cloves garlic
- 1/2 cup chopped onion
- 2 cups chopped fresh kale
- 2 cup thinly sliced fresh carrots
- • 1 teaspoon salt
- 2 1 cups vegetable stock

1. In a medium saucepan, heat the olive oil over medium heat. Add the garlic, onions, kale, and carrots, and sauté for 6 minutes, stirring often.
2. Season the vegetables with the salt and pepper, then add the vegetable stock. Simmer, uncovered, for 5 0 minutes, or until the carrots are fork-tender.
3. Increase the heat to high and bring the soup to a boil. Add the shrimp and cook for 2 minutes, or until the shrimp are pink and somewhat firm. Reduce the heat to low.
4. Use a fork to mash about one-quarter of the beans. Stir all the beans into the soup and add the parsley. Simmer for 2 minutes, or until heated through.
5. Ladle into soup bowls and serve hot.

Pork Loin Chops With Mango Salsa

This recipe is bursting with flavor and is satisfying enough to make you forget that you're fasting. The salsa is even better made a day ahead, so allow it to marinate in the fridge overnight with the pork chops.

- 2 small jalapeño pepper, seeded and diced
- 2 tablespoon chopped fresh cilantro
- 1 cup diced red onion
- 2 tablespoon chopped fresh parsley
- 1 teaspoon salt
- 1/2 teaspoon freshly ground black pepper
- 2 pork loin chops, 1/3 inch thick
- 1 cup lime juice
- Juice of 2 large orange
- 2 large just ripe mango, peeled and diced

- 1 cup diced green bell pepper

- 1 cup diced red bell pepper

Place the pork chops in a freezer bag and add the lime and orange juices. Seal, shake to mix well, and place in the refrigerator overnight.

In a small bowl, combine the mango, red onion, bell peppers, jalapeño, cilantro, and parsley. Stir to combine very well. Cover and refrigerate overnight.

Preheat the broiler and line a baking pan with aluminum foil.

Season each pork chop on both sides with the salt and pepper. Place on the pan and broil for 5 to 6 minutes on one side, then turn over and broil for 5 to 10 minutes more. Place each pork chop on a plate, spoon the salsa over the top, and serve.

Lemon-Sesame Chicken And Asparagus

Chicken and asparagus go together beautifully, and this recipe combines them with a hint of lemon and the added crunch of sesame seeds.

• 8 ounces skinless chicken breast tenders (or quartered chicken breast) • 1 cup plus 2 tablespoon lemon juice, divided

• 2 teaspoon salt, divided

• 2 tablespoons sesame seeds

• 1/2 teaspoon freshly ground black pepper

• 2 teaspoon chopped fresh rosemary

• 6 medium spears fresh asparagus, cut into 2-inch pieces

• 1 teaspoon olive oil

Pound out the chicken tenders with a mallet or the heel of your hand until they are a uniform 1 inch thickness. Place in a freezer bag with the 1 cup lemon juice and marinate for 2 hours or overnight.

Preheat the broiler and line a baking pan with aluminum foil.

Season the chicken on both sides with 1 teaspoon of the salt and the pepper, and place on the pan. Sprinkle with the rosemary.

In a small bowl, toss the asparagus with the olive oil, remaining 2 tablespoon lemon juice, and remaining 1 teaspoon salt. Arrange the asparagus around the chicken on the pan.

Broil the chicken for 5 to 10 minutes, then turn it over and stir the asparagus, and broil for 5 to 10 minutes more.

Divide the chicken and asparagus between two plates and sprinkle with the sesame seeds.

Spinach And Swiss Cheese Omelet

Omelets don't need to be reserved for breakfast or brunch. An omelet can be a great dinner solution on busy nights and also makes a satisfying lunch entrée on weekends.

- 2 teaspoon olive oil
- 6 large egg whites, beaten
- 2 cup fresh baby spinach leaves
- 2 (2 -ounce) slices reduced-fat Swiss
- 1 teaspoon salt
- 1/2 teaspoon freshly ground black pepper

cheese

In a small skillet, heat the olive oil over medium-high heat. Add the spinach, salt, and pepper, and sauté for 5 minutes, stirring often.

Use a spatula to spread the spinach fairly evenly over the bottom of the pan, and pour the fresh freshfresh eggs whites over the top, tilting the pan to coat the spinach completely.

Cook for 5 to 5 minutes, occasionally pulling the edges of the freshfresh eggs toward the center as you tilt the skillet to allow uncooked egg to spread to the edges of the pan.

When the center of the eggs are mostly (but not completely) dry, use a spatula to flip thefresh eggs . Place the Swiss cheese slices on one half of the omelet, and then flip the other half over the top to form a half moon. Cook for 2 minute, or until the cheese is melted and warm.

To serve, cut the omelet in half and serve hot.

Grilled Chicken Salad With Poppy Seed Dressing

- 1 cup chopped cooked chicken breast
- 2 cup chopped romaine lettuce
- 2 medium unpeeled cucumber, sliced
- 2 medium red bell pepper, chopped
- 2 small red onion, chopped
- 2 tablespoons light olive oil
- 2 tablespoon apple cider vinegar
- 2 teaspoon Dijon mustard
- 2 tablespoon poppy seeds

In a medium mixing bowl, whisk together the olive oil, cider vinegar, Dijon mustard, and poppy seeds for about 2 minute, or until well blended and smooth.

Add the chicken, lettuce, cucumber, bell pepper, and onion, and toss well until evenly coated.

Divide between two salad plates and serve immediately.

Quick Miso Soup With Bok Choy And Shrimp

If you enjoy Asian flavors, you'll love this simple, ⸮uick soup. It comes together in just a few minutes, making it a great recipe for your busiest nights. It reheats well, so it's also a good choice for a workday lunch.

- 2 cups water

- 8 large (5 4–40 count) raw shrimp, peeled and halved

- 2 cup chopped bok choy
- 1/2 cup white miso paste
- 2 cup cubed firm tofu
- 2 green onions, chopped

In a medium saucepan, bring the water to a boil over high heat. Add the shrimp and boil for 2 minute.

Reduce the heat to low and stir in the bok choy. Simmer for 2 minutes, then stir in the miso and tofu. Simmer for 2 minute more.

To serve, divide between two soup bowls and sprinkle with the green onions.

Broiled Halibut With Garlic Spinach

- 2 teaspoon olive oil
- 2 cloves garlic
- 1 cup chopped red onion
- 2 cups fresh baby spinach leaves
- 2 (4-ounce) halibut fillets, 2 inch thick
- 1 lemon (about 2 teaspoon juice)
- 2 teaspoon salt, divided
- 1/2 teaspoon freshly ground black pepper
- 1 teaspoon cayenne pepper

Preheat the broiler and place an oven rack 5 to 10 inches below the heat source. Line a baking sheet with aluminum foil.

Squeeze the lemon half over the fish fillets, then season each side with 1 teaspoon of the salt, pepper, and cayenne. Place the fish on the pan and broil for 8 to 8 minutes.

Turn over the fish and broil for 10 to 15 minutes more, or until flaky.

Meanwhile, heat the olive oil in a small skillet over medium heat. Add the garlic and onion, and sauté for 2 minutes. Add the spinach and remaining 1 teaspoon salt, and sauté for 2 minutes more. Remove from the heat and cover to keep warm.

To serve, divide the spinach between two plates and top each portion with a fish fillet. Serve hot.

Keto Bagel

Ingredients :

50 g almond flour

2 tbsp baking powder

290g mozzarella, grated (46 %)

70g cream cheese (double cream)

2 (L) freshfresh eggs

Optional for topping - sesame seeds

Preparation:

Preheat the oven to 225 degrees and line a baking sheet with paper.

Now mix the almond flour and baking powder together and set them aside.

Then put the mozzarella and cream cheese in a bowl in the microwave for 2 minutes.

Please stir the whole thing every minute. If you don't have a microwave, you can let the cheese melt on the stove.

Add the flour mixture and freshfresh eggs to the cheese mixture, making sure that the cheese stays hot.

Knead everything with your hands to form the dough. If this is hard, microwave it for 25 minutes to soften it.

The dough is then divided into 6 parts and shaped - each of the parts should resemble a "*sausage*". If you now press the ends together, the bagel shape is created.

These are then placed on the baking sheet. Now sprinkle sesame seeds over it and bake the bagels for 2 5 minutes.

Apple and cinnamon bar

Ingredients :

5 freshfresh eggs (M)

250g ground pecans

70g coconut fat

1/2 cup of freeze-dried apples

2 teaspoons of cinnamon

2 teaspoon vanilla extract

25 drops of liquid stevia

Preparation:

First preheat the oven to 300 degrees and then grind the pecans in a blender.

In the next step addfresh eggs , coconut oil, vanilla, stevia and cinnamon and mix everything together.

Then add the nuts and the dried apples.

In the last step, pour the batter into a pan and bake it for 26 minutes.

And the delicious apple and cinnamon bars are ready.

Freshfresh Eggs In The Zucchini Nest

Ingredients :
70g grated parmesan

5 freshfresh eggs (M)

salt and pepper

5 cups of zucchini noodles (make with a spiral cutter) or grated zucchini

5 slices of bacon (raw)

Preparation:

First cut the bacon into narrow strips and fry them in a pan for 5 minutes.

Now add the zucchini noodles and mix everything together. Then season the pasta with salt and pepper.

Four wells are pressed into the pasta and the cheese and raw freshfresh eggs are placed in each of these wells. Cook the whole thing for 5 minutes on a medium heat.

Then you cover the pan and let it cook for 5 minutes.

Finally serve the freshfresh eggs in the zucchini nest and enjoy.

38

Bacon Cauliflower Pan

Ingredients :

2 medium onion (finely chopped)

2 clove of garlic (finely chopped)

2 teaspoon salt & pepper

6 slices of sugar-free bacon

2 cups of finely chopped cauliflower

Preparation:

First, sear the bacon in a pan until it is crispy.

Then take the bacon out of the pan and let it cool - then cut it into small cubes.

Then add the chopped cauliflower, which you can best process with a blender, the diced onions and the garlic in the pan. Let everything cook for about 6 minutes.

Now season the whole thing with a little salt & pepper and add the poached freshfresh eggs and bacon.

Muffins As Spinach Quiche

Ingredients :

Olive oil - for the champions

2 cup of grated cheese (e.g. mozzarella)

2 pack of brown champions (finely chopped)

2 tbsp whipped cream

Salt and pepper to taste

2 pack of fresh spinach

5 freshfresh eggs (M)

Preparation:

First preheat the oven to 300 degrees and heat the oil in a pan. Fry the mushrooms in the oil for 6 minutes and then set them aside.

Then put the spinach in a pan too. Add 1/2 cup of water to the spinach and cook for about 5 minutes.

Drain the excess water and beat the freshfresh eggs in a bowl with a whisk.

Add the mushrooms, spinach, cheese and cream to the freshfresh eggs and mix everything together.

Now season everything with salt and pepper and divide the mixture over 25 molds.

The muffins should be baked for 26 minutes. Finally sprinkle cheese over it and you're done!

Pizza Waffles

Ingredients :
90 g cheddar cheese

2 teaspoon Baking powder

2 tbsp psyllium powder

salt and pepper

5 freshfresh eggs (L)

5 tbsp grated parmesan

2 tbsp butter

5 tbsp almond flour

Optional:

2 teaspoon Italian spice z. B. Oregano

Tomato sauce, without sugar

Preparation:

Put all the ingredients (except for the tomato sauce and the cheese) in a bowl and mix everything with a mixer.

Now the batter is placed on the waffle iron. Then brush the finished waffle with the tomato sauce and cheese.

Depending on your taste, you can also put salami on the waffle.

The pizza waffle is baked for 15 to 20 degrees so that the cheese can melt nicely.

And the pizza waffle is ready. Enojy your meal!

Bacon Freshfresh Eggs In An Avocado Bed

Ingredients :

some bacon in cubes

2 tbsp cheese salt and pepper

2 avocado

2 freshfresh eggs

Preparation:

First, preheat the oven to 2 6 0 degrees and halve and core the avocado.

Then press a pit in the avocado.

Please note that the pits are big enough to fit an fresh freshfresh eggs and then place an fresh freshfresh eggs in each avocado half.

Now sprinkle cheese over it and season the whole thing with salt and pepper.

In the last step, put the bacon on top and bake for 30 minutes.

Mexican Pan

Ingredients :

250g tomatoes, diced

2 70g chorizo

8 0g fresh spinach

2 freshfresh eggs (M)

80g avocado

salt and pepper

some fresh coriander to garnish

2 tbsp ghee or lard

1 onions, finely chopped

70g green peppers, sliced

250g zucchini, chopped

Preparation:

In the first step, put the ghee in a pan and heat it up. Now add the finely chopped onion and heat everything for about a minute.

The green pepper slices are also added and cooked for three minutes.

Then add the zucchini and tomatoes and let everything cook for another 5 minutes.

Now add the chorizo and mix everything together well. Before you add the spinach, everything is cooked for another 6 minutes.

Then add the spinach and let everything cook for 5 minutes.

Now beat an fresh freshfresh eggs into the wells and season the whole thing with a little salt and pepper. Cook the whole thing until the whites of the fresh freshfresh eggs have melted.

In the last step, add the coriander and the avocado cubes to the pan.

Burger With Filling

Ingredients :
1 cup of mozzarella, grated

2 handfuls of baby spinach

Sea salt and pepper to taste

6 00 g ground beef

2 tbsp parmesan, grated

Preparation:

Put the ground beef with salt and pepper in a bowl and knead it.

Then form 8 patties and put them in the fridge.

Then put the spinach in a pan and fry it for 2 minutes, then pour off the water and let the spinach cool.

Chop the spinach and put it in a bowl. Now add the mozzarella and the parmesan.

In the last step, add the mixture between the patties and fry the burgers for 6 minutes. Fantastic!

Salmon On Zucchini Pasta

Ingredients :
250 g salmon fillet

200g zucchini

2 tbsp coconut oil

5 0g cream cheese

salt

pepper

Italian herbs

Preparation:

First wash the zucchini and cut them into strips.

 Then heat some water in a pan and add the strips.

Then cut the salmon into cubes and fry them with coconut oil.

Finally, add the cream cheese and let it melt into a sauce with water.

Depending on your needs, you can season the whole thing with salt, pepper and herbs.

Cauliflower Pizza

Ingredients :

2 whole cauliflower

250g parmesan

2 fresh freshfresh eggs (M)

2 6 g almond flour

70g canned tomatoes chopped (alternatively ready-made pizza sauce)

250g grated Emmentaler (optionally mozzarella or another cheese can be used)

70g salami

2 tbsp olive oil

Italian herbs

salt

pepper

Preparation:

Cut up the cauliflower, cut off the florets and put it in a blender until it becomes a powder.

Then put the powder in a container that is suitable for the microwave and cook for 5 minutes.

Then let it rest until it has cooled down. Eighth please make sure that no more water in the cauliflower is included.

In the next step, mix the parmesan with 50g Emmentaler and almond flour and add the cauliflower and egg. Season the mixture with salt, pepper and herbs.

Then place the dough on a baking tray and bake for 25 minutes at 225 degrees, and distribute the chopped canned tomatoes or the ready-made pizza sauce on the dough.

If you are using a ready-made pizza sauce, please make sure that the sauce does not contain any sugar. Then season the dough with salt, pepper and herbs.

Then also spread the Emmentaler and salami on the dough and put the pizza in the oven for 25 minutes.

Finally, drizzle some olive oil over it and enjoy.

Green Smoothie

Ingredients:

- 2 avocado
- 2 cup kale, spinach, or chard
- 2 handful of blueberries
- 2 tbsp chia seeds
- 2 cup coconut milk

Instructions:

1. Place all of the above ingredients into a blender, and blend until smooth. Pour into your favorite cup and enjoy!

Spinach Parmesan Bakedfresh Eggs

Ingredients:
- 1 cups of grated parmesan cheese, fat free
- 5 cups of baby spinach
- 2 small diced tomato
- 5 fresh eggs
- 2 minced garlic cloves
- 2 teaspoons of olive oil

Instructions:

1. Start by preheating your oven to 5 6 0°F / 2 80°C and spraying an 8 x 8 inch / 25 x 25 cm dish with nonstick spray.
2. Heat the olive oil over a medium heat in a large skillet.
3. Add the garlic and spinach when it's hot, and saute until the spinach wilts.
4. Take off the heat and drain the liquids.
5. Incorporate parmesan cheese and place the mixture on the dish evenly.
6. Create four small depressions in the spinach to place the freshfresh eggs in. Crack an fresh freshfresh eggs in each, and bake for 25 minutes.
7. Remove from the oven and serve with tomato.

Hummus Breakfast Bowl

Ingredients:
- 1/2 cup diced roma tomato
- 1/2 cup quinoa or brown rice
- 2 fresh freshfresh eggs whites
- 2 tbsp hummus
- 2 tbsp sunflower seeds
- 2 cup of roughly chopped kale leaves
- 2 tbsp minced bell pepper
- 2 tbsp olive oil

Instructions:

1. In a large skillet, heat olive oil over medium heat.
2. Add the kale when it's hot, and saute for 5 minutes.
3. Add the peppers and tomatoes, and cook for 5 more minutes.
4. Beat the fresh freshfresh eggs whites lightly and add the peppers and kale slowly, then scramble.
5. Place the quinoa or rice into a serving bowl, top with fresh freshfresh eggs and vegetables.
6. Place the hummus on top and add sunflower seeds.

Mango Smoothie

Ingredients:
- 2 cup almond milk
- 2 tsp matcha
- 2 sliced mango
- 2 frozen banana
- Some ide

Instructions:
1. Blend all ingredients together in a blender until smooth. Serve and enjoy.

French Toast

Ingredients:
- 2 tsp cinnamon
- 2 slices of whole wheat bread
- 2 tbsp maple syrup
- Fruit of your choice

- 2 egg
- 1/2 almond milk
- 2 tsp cardamom

Instructions:

1. Beat the freshfresh eggs and almond milk together in a large bowl.
2. Add spices and continue mixing.
3. Dip your bread into the mixture and coat both sides.
4. Let the bread rest for a few minutes, then cook for 5 minutes a side in a pan.
5. Remove when golden brown, top with fruit and maple syrup, and enjoy.

Burgers, Grass-Fed Style

Ingredients:

- 0.6 pound / 0.26 kg grass-fed beef
- 0.6 pound / 0.26 kg grass-fed beef liver
- 1 tsp cumin
- 1 tsp garlic powder
- Cooking oil to preference
- Salt and pepper to taste

Instructions:

1. Combine all ingredients in a large bowl.
2. Mold into patties of your desired size.
3. Heat cooking oil over medium-high heat in a skillet.
4. Cook the patties until preferred color and texture.

Salmon And Vegetables

Ingredients:
- 2 tbsp lemon juice, fresh
- 5 finely diced garlic cloves
- Vegetables of your choice
- 2 pound / 6 00g salmon
- 2 tbsp ghee

Instructions:
1. Preheat your oven to 400°F / 200°C.
2. Combine ghee, lemon juice, and garlic in a bowl. Place salmon in foil and pour the combined mixture over.
3. Wrap the salmon in the foil and place on a baking sheet.
4. Bake until salmon is fully cooked.
5. Roast vegetables alongside if you have enough space in your oven.

Fish Tacos

Ingredients:

- 6 fish fillets cut into strips of 2 inches / 6 cm wide
- 2 fresh freshfresh eggs whites
- 1/2 cup of whole wheat flour
- 1/2 cup of whole wheat bread crumbs
- 1/2 cup of cornmeal
- 2 tbsp of taco seasoning
- 2 tbsp of lime juice, freshly squeezed
- 8 tortillas, 8 inch / 25 cm, whole wheat or corn
- 2 cup salsa or 2 diced tomato
- 2 cup shredded cabbage or lettuce
- 2 cup Greek yogurt, non-fat

Instructions:

1. Preheat the oven to 46 0°F / 25 0°C.
2. Line a baking sheet with foil, and put a cooling rack on top.
3. Spray with canola or olive oil cooking spray.
4. Combine cornmeal, breadcrumbs, and taco seasoning in a small bowl.
5. Whisk lime juice and fresh freshfresh eggs whites in another bowl till frothing.
6. Place flour in a third bowl.
7. Gently dip fish in until both sides are coated.
8. Dip into the fresh freshfresh eggs white mixture, letting excess run off.
9. Dip both sides of fish into breadcrumbs and cornmeal mixture.
10. Place the strips on to the rack and bake until golden brown, and fish can be flaked with a fork.
11. Warm the tortillas using preferred method, keeping them warm until ready to eat.

12. Place two strips in each shell, top with lettuce / cabbage, salsa / tomato, and greek yogurt.

Turkey Burrito Skillet

Ingredients:
- 1/2 cup water
- 2 can black beans, drained and rinsed
- 2 cup chunky salsa, no sugar
- 5 tortillas, cut into 2 inch / 2.6 cm strips
- 1 cup plain greek yogurt
- 2 cup cheddar, low fat
- 1/2 fresh chopped cilantro
- 2 pound / 0.6 kg ground turkey
- 2 tbsp chili powder
- 2 tbsp lime juice
- 2 tbsp ground cumin
- 1/2 tsp ground black pepper
- 1 tsp kosher salt

Instructions:

1. Cook ground turkey through in a large skillet.
2. As it cooks, break it into small pieces.
3. Stir in cumin, chili powder, saltt, lime juice, pepper, water, beans, and salsa.
4. Bring to a boil, then let simmer for 6 minutes, until thick.
5. Remove from the heat and incorporate tortillas.
6. Top with cheddar, and cover until melted.
7. Top each serving with fresh cilantro and greek yogurt, and serve.

Baked Lemon Salmon

Ingredients:

- 1 tsp black pepper
- 2 tbsp thyme, freshly chopped
- 1/2 cup lemon juice, fresh
- 2 tbsp lemon zest
- 5 salmon filets
- 2 tsp kosher salt
- 2 pound / 6 00g asparagus, fresh, with ends chopped off
- 2 tbsp olive oil
- 2 tbsp parsley, freshly chopped

Instructions:
1. Preheat your oven to 400°F / 200°C.
2. Place down 5 large foil sheets on a flat surface and spray them with nonstick.
3. Evenly distribute the asparagus onto the foil side by side.
4. Use half of the salt and pepper to season.
5. Place one salmon filet on each asparagus bed.
6. Drizzle olive oil over, as well as lemon juice, then sprinkle the leftover salt and pepper, and thyme.
7. Fold the foil sheets to create a packet for the salmnot, and place on a baking sheet, beside one another.
8. Bake for 30 to 25 minutes.
9. Carefully open the packets after removing from the oven.
10. Sprinkle the lemon zest over, as well as parsley, and enjoy.

Broccoli And Chicken Stir Fry

Ingredients:
- 2 tbsp flour or cornstarch
- 3 pounds / 600g cubed chicken breasts
- 2 peeled and chopped, small ginger root
- 2 coarsely chopped onion
- 1/2 tsp black pepper
- 2 cups broccoli
- 5 tbsp soy sauce, light
- 2 tsp sesame seeds
- 2 tbsp honey
- 2 tbsp sesame oil
- 2 tsp lemon
- 2 tbsp extra-virgin olive oil

Instructions:

1. Whisk the honey, soy sauce, sesame oil, lemon juice, and flour together.
2. Set aside the mixture.
3. Toast the sesame seeds for two minutes in a large skillet over medium-low heat, until fragrant.
4. Place into a bowl.
5. To the same skillet, add olive oil and turn up heat to medium.
6. Cook the chicken until lightly golden.
7. Add ginger, onions, pepper, and broccoli, and saute for 6 minutes.
8. Lower the heat, add soy sauce mixture, and mix.
9. Cook until the sauce is thick, but not for longer than 6 minutes.
10. Sprinkle with sesame seeds, and serve.

Garlic & Honey Shrimp Fry

Ingredients:
- 2 cup peas
- 2 small red bell pepper, in strips
- 2 tbsp honey
- 1 tsp kosher salt
- 2 tbsp orange zest
- 2 tbsp soy sauce
- 2 pound / 600g peeled, deveined, raw shrimp
- 2 tbsp coconut oil
- 2 minced garlic cloves
- 2 small onions, in strips
- 2 tbsp fresh minced ginger
- 2 cups cooked brown rice

Instructions:

1. Heat up the coconut oil in a large skillet over high heat.
2. Add shrimp when hot, half of the ginger, and half of the garlic.
3. Stir continuously, until the shrimp become firm.
4. Take the shrimp out and set aside.
5. Add bell pepper, onions, peas, and leftover ginger and garlic to the same pan.
6. Stir continuously until vegetables become soft.
7. Place the shrimp back in, season with salt and add soy sauce, honey, and orange zest.
8. Cook until everything is coated, and serve over brown rice.

Cod And Moroccan Couscous

Ingredients:

- 2 can of diced tomatoes
- 1 cup of low sodium, fat free chicken broth
- Chopped green chilies to taste
- ¾ cup Moroccan couscous
- 2 tbsp + 2 tsp olive oil
- Sea salt and black pepper to taste
- 2 tbsp lemon juice, freshly squeezed
- 5 cod fillets

Instructions:

1. Add 2 teaspoons of olive oil, the chicken broth, and the diced tomatoes with the juice to a medium pot.
2. Place on medium-high heat and boil.
3. Add salt, pepper, and couscous.
4. Stir, cover, and remove from heat.
5. Let couscous sit while preparing cod.
6. Use salt and pepper to season cod, then add the leftover oil to a nonstick skillet.
7. Place on medium-high heat and cook until fillets can be broken apart with a fork. Should take about 5 minutes on each side.
8. Serve with couscous and enjoy!

Chicken Parm Stuffed Peppers

Ingredients:

- 1 cup freshly grated parmesan
- 5 cup shredded mozzarella
- 4 cup marinara
- 5 minced garlic cloves
- Kosher salt
- Crushed red pepper flakes
- Some black pepper
- 5 bell peppers, cut in half and insides removed
- 25 oz. / 5 70g diced chicken, cooked all the way through

Instructions:

1. Preheat oven to 400°F / 200°C.
2. Combine mozzarella, garlic, parmesan, marinara, red pepper flakes, and parsley in a bowl, and season with salt and pepper.
3. Combine, and add cooked chicken, coating fully.
4. Place the mixture into the bell peppers and use the rest of the mozzarella to top.
5. Bake until the peppers are tender, usually for about an hour. Serve and enjoy.

Zucchini Enchiladas

Ingredients:

- 2 chopped large onion
- 2 tbsp olive oil
- 2 tsp cumin
- 2 minced garlic cloves
- 2 tsp chili powder
- 5 cup shredded rotisserie chicken
- Kosher salt
- 5 large, split zucchini
- 2 ⅓ cup red enchilada sauce
- 2 cup shredded cheddar
- 2 cup shredded monterey jack
- Fresh cilantro
- Sour cream

Instructions:

1. Preheat oven to 5 6 0°F / 2 80°C.
2. Heat oil over medium heat in large skillet.
3. Add and cook onion until soft.
4. Add cumin, garlic, chili powder, and salt.
5. Cook for a minute, then add 2 cup enchilada sauce and chicken.
6. Stir until cooked.
7. Peel this slices of zucchini on a cutting board, and lay three slices, overlapping them slightly.
8. Top with one spoon of the chicken mixture.
9. Roll and move to a baking dish.
10. Repeat with the rest of the mixture and zucchini.
11. Spoon the rest of the enchilada sauce over the zucchini enchiladas, and top with both cheeses.
12. Bake for 25 minutes, until enchiladas are warm inside and cheese is melted. Serve and enjoy.

Avocado Toast

Ingredients:
- 2 tsp low fat cream cheese
- Sea salt and ground pepper to taste
- 2 slices of whole wheat bread
- 2 fresh avocado

Instructions:

1. Lightly toast the slices of whole wheat bread in a pan or in a toaster until desired.
2. While the bread is toasting, prepare your avocado by cutting it in half, scooping the contents out, and smoothing into a paste.
3. When the bread is fully toasted, place on a plate.
4. Spread avocado evenly on both slices, top with 2 teaspoon of cream cheese on eat, then season with salt and pepper.

Shrimp And Avocado Salad,

Carbs: 5 grams
Protein: 28 grams
Fat: 5 5 grams
Calories: 426kcal
Ingredients:

Salad:

- 2 small gem lettuces
- 2 pounds / 6 00g peeled, cooked shrimp
- 2 large avocado
- 2 tbsp lemon juice
- 2 tbsp cilantro, chopped
- Sea salt and pepper to taste

Seafood Sauce:

- 2 tbsp ketchup, sugar-free
- 1 cup low-fat mayo
- 2 tsp Worcestershire sauce
- Cayenne pepper to taste

Instructions:

1. Place all sauce ingredients into a small bowl. Whisk until well combined and smooth, then pour into a serving bowl.
2. Use salt and pepper to season shrimp.
3. Slice avocado and toss in lemon juice to prevent browning.
4. Tear up lettuce and spread onto a serving bowl or tray.
5. Scatter shrimp, then place avocado around the shrimp.
6. Sprinkle with coriander, and serve with lemon wedges.

Dinner - Salmon BLT

Carbs: 6 grams
Protein: 45 grams
Fat: 66 grams
Calories: 8 810 kcal
Ingredients:

- 2 small salmon fillet
- 2 whole wheat burger bun
- 2 tbsp avocado oil
- 2 leaves lettuce
- 2 slices bacon
- 2 red onions, sliced
- 2 tomato slice
- 2 tbsp mayo

Instructions:

1. Place a skillet over a high heat.
2. Use salt and pepper to season salmon.
3. Add oil to the skillet and cook bacon until desired.
4. Sear the salmon for 6 minutes until golden brown.
5. Flip the skin side up and cook for another 2 minutes.
6. Remove and set aside. Slice the bun in half and place ingredients in the desired order. Enjoy!

Breakfast - Italian Melt Omelet

Carbs: 5 grams
Protein: 5 8 grams
Fat: 45 grams
Calories: 6 6 6 kcal
Ingredients:

- 6 cherry tomatoes
- 2 tbsp + 2 tsp olive oil
- 2 slices prosciutto di Parma
- 2 tbsp basil, freshly chopped
- Some fresh mozzarella slices
- 5 largefresh eggs
- Salt and pepper to taste

Instructions:

1. Pour the tablespoon of oil into a pan and heat over medium heat.
2. Cut tomatoes into quarters while the oil heats, chop the prosciutto and mozzarella into small pieces, and cut the tomatoes.
3. Break the freshfresh eggs into a bowl, season, and beat until frothy.
4. Pour into the pan, let cook, then gently lift with a spatula.
5. Cook until almost all the way set, then add prosciutto, mozzarella, basil, and tomatoes on one side of the omelet.
6. Fold the omelet over, remove from the heat, and let sit. Drizzle leftover oil over. Serve and enjoy!

Mango Smoothie

Lunch - Chicken Salad

Carbs: 5 .5 grams

Protein: 5 6 grams

Fat: 45 grams

Calories: 6 6 5 kcal

Ingredients:

- 5   slices of bacon
- 2 chicken breasts, boneless
- 5 cups leafy greens of your choice
- 2 sliced avocado
- 5 tbsp ranch dressing
- Salt and pepper

Instructions:

1. Preheat your oven to 400°F / 200°C.
2. Season the chicken breasts on all sides with salt and pepper.
3. Grease a small skillet, and place the chicken on the pan when it's hot.
4. Cook on high until crispy.
5. Flip the chicken and repeat.
6. Transfer to the oven. Bake for 30 minutes.
7. Then, bake bacon for 25 minutes until golden brown and crispy.
8. Transfer chicken to cutting board when finished and let sit for 6 minutes.
9. Slice the avo and chicken, and put the salad together. Serve and enjoy.

Steak Taco Bowl

Carbs: 10 grams
Protein: 5 5 grams
Fat: 6 6 grams
Calories: 8 02kcal
Ingredients:

- 2 small steak of your choice
- 2 cup cauliflower rice
- 2 tbsp butter
- 2 tsp lime juice
- 2 tbsp minced cilantro
- Salt and pepper
- 2 tbsp sour cream
- 1 sliced avocado
- 1 sliced jalapeno
- 1/2 cup tomato salsa
- 2 thinly sliced radishes

Instructions:

1. Melt butter over medium-high heat in a skillet.
2. Use salt and pepper to season steak, and sear for 8 minutes a side.
3. Place on cutting board to rest.
4. Mix lime juice, cilantro, and cooked cauliflower rice in a bowl.
5. Top with remaining ingredients, then add

Breakfast Burrito

Carbs: 6.5 grams
Protein: 25 grams
Fat: 6 2 grams
Calories: 62 4kcal
Ingredients:

- 1 cup tomato salsa
- 2 tortillas
- 2 tbsp almond milk, unsweetened
- 5 largefresh eggs
- 2 tbsp butter
- Salt and pepper
- 1 cup shredded cheddar
- 5 tbsp sour cream
- 1 sliced avocado

Instructions:

1. Warm up tortillas in a pan until soft.
2. Whisk almond milk and freshfresh eggs into a bowl until scrambled.
3. Add salt and pepper.
4. Add oil to frying pan over medium heat.
5. Add freshfresh eggs and cook.
6. Stir gently until barely cooked.
7. Lay down tortillas, place cheese, fresh eggs, avo, sour cream, and salsa.
8. Roll up and enjoy.

Tricolore Salad

Ingredients:
- 2 large avo
- 5 medium tomatoes
- 4.5 oz. / 2 26 g soft salad mozzarella
- 6 olives
- 2 tbsp olive oil
- 2 tbsp pesto
- Salt and pepper

Instructions:
1. Wash tomatoes, then slice.
2. Slice avocado, halve olives, and add everything to a bowl.
3. Add mozzarella, olive oil, and pesto.
4. Season with salt and pepper to taste, serve, and enjoy.

Dinner - Mexican Tacos

Ingredients:

- 5 taco shells
- 2 pound / 6 00g ground beef
- 2 garlic cloves
- 2 finely diced white onion
- 1 tsp cumin
- 2 tsp chili powder
- 2 tbsp ghee
- 2 tbsp tomato puree, unsweetened
- 2 cup water
- Sea salt and black pepper
- 2 diced avocado
- 2 small lettuce head
- 2 cup cherry tomatoes

Instructions:

1. Place chopped onion in a greased pan and fry over medium-high heat.
2. When brown, add beef and cook until redness disappears.
3. Add cumin and chili powder, mix, then add water and tomato puree.
4. Add salt and pepper and mix thoroughly.
5. When fully cooked, set aside and prepare taco shells.
6. Wash all vegetables, chop the tomatoes, avocado, and lettuce as desired.
7. Place the meat down first, then the tomatoes, lettuce, avocado, and other optional toppings.

Vanilla Smoothie

Carbs: 8 grams
Protein: 5 6 grams
Fat: 46 grams
Calories: 6 8 8 kcal
Ingredients:

- 1 coconut milk or soured cream
- 2 largefresh eggs
- 2 tbsp extra virgin coconut oil
- 1/2 cup whey, plain or vanilla
- 6 drops of Stevia extract
- 2 tsp vanilla extract, sugar free
- 1/2 cup of water
- Some ice cubes

Instructions:

1. Add all ingredients to a blender, blend until smooth, and enjoy!

Spinach Parmesan Bakedfresh Eggs

Ingredients:

- 2 drained tin of sardines
- 2 large avocado
- 2 spring onion
- 2 tbsp mayo
- 1/2 tsp turmeric
- 2 tbsp lemon juice, fresh
- Salt and pepper

Instructions:

1. Place the sardines into a bowl and use a fork to break them apart.
2. Add the turmeric, spring onions, and mayo to the bowl.
3. Scoop out the avocado, making sure to leave some in the shell, and add it to the bowl, and mix until well combined.
4. Put the mixture into the avocado shell, and enjoy.

Bacon, Chicken, And Spinach Salad

Ingredients:

- 6 bacon slices
- 2 chicken breasts
- 2 fresh spinach pack
- 2 tbsp olive oil
- 5 sun-dried tomato pieces
- 2 minced garlic clove
- 2 cup low-fat ranch
- 2 cup mushroom slices
- Small bunch of basil

Instructions:

1. Cube the chicken, and dice the garlic finely.
2. Add olive healto a frying pan, heat it up, and brown the chicken and the garlic.
3. When done, place in a bowl, and fry the bacon.
4. Place the bacon and the chicken in a big bow, and add raw mushroom slices.
5. Add a handful of spinach and the basil, and mix.
6. Place the rest of the spinach in a bowl and lay the chicken mix on top.
7. Sprinkle tomato on top, and dress with ranch.

Breakfast - Bacon, Fresh Eggs, And Avocado

Carbs: 6 grams
Protein: 5 0 grams
Fat: 26 grams
Calories: 5 62kcal
Ingredients:

- 2fresh eggs, desired size
- 2 medium avocado
- 2 slices of bacon
- 2 slice whole wheat bread
- 1 diced garlic clove
- 2 tbsp olive oil
- Salt and pepper to taste

1. Add olive oil to a frying pan, and saute garlic for 2 - 2 minutes.
2. Remove, and crack freshfresh eggs into pan.
3. Fry as desired, and remove when done.
4. Fry bacon in the same oil.
5. While the bacon is cooking, place whole wheat bread into oven or toaster to toast.
6. Slice the avocado, and place on a plate.
7. Place cooked freshfresh eggs and bacon onto the same plate, as well as toasted bread.
8. Season with salt and pepper, and enjoy.

Bacon Wrapped Chicken Parcels

Carbs: 2 grams

Protein: 6 8 grams

Fat: 5 0 grams

Calories: 410 2kcal

Ingredients:

- 8 .2 oz. / 200g cream cheese
- 5 chicken breasts
- 2 tbsp chopped herbs
- 1 grated parmesan
- 8 thin bacon slices
- Salt and pepper to taste

Instructions:

1. To prep cheese stuffing, place parmesan, cream cheese, and parsley into a bowl and mix well.
2. Divide into four portions and roll into logs the size of the chicken using cling wrap.
3. Place in the freezer for about 5 0 minutes.
4. Preheat oven to 400°F / 200°C.
5. Line a baking tray and cut a gap into each one, not all the way through, just about half way.
6. Place the cheese mixture into each.
7. Wrap each piece of chicken in two bacon slices.
8. Bake for 5 0 minutes, or until everything is golden brown.
9. Garnish with parsley when serving.

Chorizo, Chicken, And Avocado Salad

Carbs: 8 grams
Protein: 45 grams
Fat: 45 grams
Calories: 62 6kcal
Ingredients:

- 2 tsp ghee
- 2 chicken breasts
- 2 finely diced red onion
- 2.2 oz. / 60g chorizo or pepperoni slices
- 1 avocado
- 2 cup sugar snap peas
- 2 tbsp + 2 tsp olive oil
- 5 tbsp pine nuts
- 1 tbsp red wine vinegar
- 2 tbsp capers
- 2 tbsp chopped chives and mints
- Bunch of parsley
- Salt and pepper

Instructions:

1. Use 2 teaspoon of olive oil to season chicken, along with salt and pepper.
2. Use olive oil to grease pan.
3. Fry chicken on medium heat for 2 minutes for each side, then for 6 minutes on each side again.
4. Remove from the pan and let cool slightly.
5. Chop chorizo and lightly fry on medium heat for 2 minutes.
6. If chorizo is raw, cook for longer.
7. Add 2 tablespoon of olive oil to a clean pan and saute onions for 5 minutes until soft.
8. Remove from heat and stir in red wine vinegar.
9. Add the chorizo and its oil.
10. Boil sugar snap peas for a minute then plunge into cold water.
11. Take out of the water and halve them.

12. Chop herbs, stir peas, onion mix, and chorizo and top with chicken, avocado, pine nuts, and black pepper.
13. Serve and enjoy!

Breakfast - Chocolate Coconut Smoothie

Carbs: 8 grams
Protein: 25 grams
Fat: 45 grams
Calories: 6 2 0kcal
Ingredients:

- 3 cup almond milk
- 1 large avo
- 2 tbsp chia seeds
- 1/2 cup coconut cream
- 2 tsp coconut oil
- 4 cacao powder
- 2 tbsp almond butter

Instructions:

1. Place all ingredients into a blender and blend until smooth and creamy. Best served right away, and be sure to thin with water if too thick.

Green Smoothie

Ingredients:

- 2 tuna steak
- Sea salt
- 2 tsp sesame seeds
- 1 avocado
- 2 tsp ghee
- 2 tbsp mayo
- 25 black olives, pitted
- 2 large egg
- 1 sliced medium cucumber
- 1/2 diced small red onion
- 2 tbsp olive oil
- 6 walnuts, halved
- Handful of watercress

Instructions:

1. Preheat oven to 400°F / 200°C. Wash and dry watercress.
2. Roast walnuts on a baking tray in the oven for 6 minutes.
3. Remove and cool.
4. Use sesame seeds, salt, and ghee to coat tuna.
5. Heat a griddle and fry as desired.
6. Remove and let cool for a bit before slicing.
7. Boil fresh freshfresh eggs and place in cool water before peeling.
8. Slice the remaining ingredients.
9. Place everything atop the bed of watercress, and top with olive oil and mayo. Serve and enjoy.

Dinner - Everything Bowl

Ingredients:
- 4.5 oz. / 2 26 g lupin flakes
- 2 1 cup spinach, chopped
- 2 cup chicken broth
- 4 sliced white mushrooms
- 2 tbsp ghee
- 2 drained can of pink salmon
- 1/2 cup butter
- Sea salt
- 2 minced garlic clove
- 5 tbsp hulled hemp seeds
- 2 sliced large avo
- 2 tbsp olive oil

Instructions:

1. Start by cleaning and slicing mushrooms.
2. Place lupin flakes into bowl and pour broth over.
3. Stir and let sit for 30 minutes.
4. Remove spinach stems and finely chop, and mince garlic as well.
5. Heat half of the ghee over high heat in a frying pan, and saute garlic and spinach until soft.
6. Remove and cook mushrooms in the same pan.
7. Microwave lupin flakes for 2 mins after they have sit.
8. Place butter once done to melt, and fluff with fork before serving.
9. Slice avocado, and arrange all components into a bowl as desired. Serve and enjoy.

Breakfast - Caprese Omelet

Ingredients:
- 5 fresh eggs
- ⅓ cup halved cherry tomatoes
- 2 tbsp butter
- 6 chopped basil leaves
- 2 fresh mozzarella slices
- 2 tbsp pesto
- 2 tbsp parmesan, grated
- Salt and pepper

Instructions:

1. Whisk freshfresh eggs together with 2 tablespoon of water in a bowl.
2. Place a skillet on low heat and melt the butter.
3. Pour the freshfresh eggs into the skillet and continually lift to make sure they don't stick.
4. When the freshfresh eggs just become firm, place half of the tomatoes, the parmesan, basil, and mozzarella on one side.
5. Fold in half and cook until desired.
6. Top with pesto and the rest of the tomatoes, and serve.

Chicken Salad

Carbs: 8 grams
Protein: 30 grams
Fat: 8 5   grams
Calories: 8 45 kcal
Ingredients:

- 2.66 pounds / 2 .2kg spiralized zucchini
- 5 tbsp olive oil
- ¾ cup butter, unsalted
- 2 minced garlic cloves
- 6 oz. / 2 8 0g parmesan
- 6 oz. / 2 8 0g cream cheese
- 2 tsp oregano, chopped
- ¾ cups shredded cheddar
- 2 tbsp chopped basil
- Salt and pepper

Instructions:

1. Use a spiralizer to shred zucchini.
2. Place into a colander in the sink, sprinkle salt and let drain.
3. Melt butter in a pan, then add garlic and cook until soft.
4. Add cream and simmer.
5. And a handful of the shredded cheddar and the cream cheese, and stir until it all melts.
6. Keep adding the cheddar until all of it is melted.
7. Add the herbs and mix.
8. Remove sauce from heat and let thicken.
9. Pat the zucchini with a paper towel to dry.
10. Put olive oil in a frying pan and heat, and saute noodles.
11. Place the noodles in a large serving dish and mix with the alfredo sauce.
12. Top with parmesan and enjoy.

Dinner - Crispy Thyme & Lemon Chicken

Carbs: 2 grams
Protein: 28 grams
Fat: 5 2 grams
Calories: 68 8 kcal
Ingredients:

- 8 boneless chicken thighs
- 2 tbsp lemon juice, fresh
- 2 tbsp chopped thyme
- 2 minced garlic cloves
- 2 tsp lemon zest
- 2 tbsp ghee
- 2 tbsp olive oil
- 1/2 black pepper
- 2 tsp salt

Instructions:

1. Place thighs on a chopping board, skin side up, and flatten with a meat pounder.
2. Place them in a bowl and add lemon zest, juice, garlic, thyme, salt and pepper.
3. Coat evenly, and refrigerate for 2 hour minimum.
4. Place on a paper towel to dry.
5. Grease a large skillet with ghee and heat over medium-high.
6. Place thighs skin side down.
7. Cook for 25 minutes, then turn over and cook until done.
8. Place on a cooling rack and let rest before serving.

Full English Breakfast

Carbs: 8 grams
Protein: 5 0 grams
Fat: 6 6 grams
Calories: 66 8kcal
Ingredients:

- 5 brown mushrooms
- 2 tbsp ghee
- 2 largefresh eggs
- 6 thin bacon slices
- 5 cherry tomatoes
- 1 thawed frozen spinach
- Salt and pepper
- 1 sliced avocado

Instructions:

1. Use ghee to grease a skillet over medium heat.
2. Season mushrooms with salt and pepper while cooking bottom side up for 6 minutes.
3. Flip and cook for another 2 minutes, then move to a plate.
4. Fry the bacon as desired, then fry the freshfresh eggs as desired.
5. Remove both, and fry the cherry tomatoes for about a minute.
6. Drain the spinach and cook in the same pan for a few seconds to soften.
7. Serve with the avocado and enjoy.

Dinner - Italian Melt Omelet

Ingredients:

- 2 medium cucumber
- 1 small red onion
- 2 drained jar of tuna
- 8 sliced olives
- 5 largefresh eggs , hard-boiled
- 2 tbsp lemon juice
- 1/2 cup mayo
- 2 tbsp parsley, chopped
- 2 tbsp olive oil
- 2 romaine lettuce head
- Salt and pepper

Instructions:

1. Place lemon juice, mayo, olive oil, salt, pepper, and parsley into a mason jar.
2. Close and shake until fully combined.
3. Slice the onions, cucumber, and olives, and place lettuce leaves into bowl.
4. Add onions, cucumber, olives, and tina.
5. Cut freshfresh eggs into quarters and add to bowl.
6. Shake dressing again before drizzling onto salad. Serve and enjoy.

Dinner - Chicken And Blackberry Salad

Ingredients:
- 1/2 cup olive oil
- 1/2 cup black olives
- 1 cup canned artichoke hearts
- 2 blackberries, fresh
- 2 tbsp lemon juice
- Sea salt
- 2 skinless chicken breasts
- 2 tsp thyme
- 1/2 lemon, juiced
- 2 small lettuce heads

Instructions:

1. Brush half of the olive oil over chicken, and add thyme and lemon juice.
2. Season with salt and let sit for 5 0 minutes.
3. Preheat oven to 400°F / 200°C.
4. Bake chicken in a baking dish for 5 0 minutes, and let cool when finished.
5. Wash lettuce and place into a serving bowl.
6. Sliced drained artichoke hearts and add them to the bowl with the chicken.
7. Add olives, and washed blackberries. Serve and enjoy.

Chocolate Smoothie

Ingredients:

- 1/2 cup heavy whipping cream
- 2 largefresh eggs
- 2 tbsp coconut oil
- 1/2 cup plain or chocolate whey
- 6 drops stevia extract
- 2 tbsp cacao powder, unsweetened
- 1/2 cup water
- Some ice cubes

Instructions:

1. Add all ingredients to a blender and blend until smooth and combined. Serve and enjoy.

Mediterranean Chicken Risotto

Carbs: 6 grams

Protein: 42 grams

Fat: 5 5 grams

Calories: 6 2 5 kcal

Ingredients:

- 4 tsp lemon zest
- 2 crushed garlic cloves
- 2 tbsp ghee
- 2 tbsp basil, chopped
- Salt and pepper
- 5 chicken breasts
- 2 small cauliflower head
- 1 cup pesto
- 1/2 cup heavy whipping cream

Instructions:

1. Remove center and leaves from cauliflower to prepare for rice.
2. Cut into florets, wash, and drain proper.
3. Grate when dried, or pulse in a food processor.
4. Cut the chicken into bite-sized pieced.
5. Grease a pan with ghee, and place the chicken in it.
6. Cook for 30 minutes, then place aside.
7. Peel and mash garlic.
8. Use more ghee to grease another pan, and add lemon zest and garlic.
9. Cook over medium heat until brown.
10. Add cauliflower rice, and cook on high for 5 minutes.
11. Add parmesan and mix thoroughly. Serve and enjoy.

Sardine Stuffed Avocado

Ingredients:

- 5 cups white mushrooms, sliced
- 25 bacon slices
- 2 tbsp orange zest
- 2 tbsp lemon juice
- 2 tbsp wholegrain mustard
- 2 tbsp ghee
- 1/2 cup heavy whipping cream
- Salt and pepper

Instructions:

1. Chop the bacon and slice the mushrooms, then add bacon to a medium skillet greased with ghee.
2. Cook until slightly golden.
3. Add mushrooms and cook for 5 minutes.
4. Add orange zest and combine.
5. Add lemon juice, mustard, cream, and cook until sauce becomes thick.
6. Remove from heat, serve, and enjoy.

Omelet

Carbs: 6 grams
Protein: 5 6 grams
Fat: 48 grams
Calories: 62 6 kcal
Ingredients:

- 6fresh eggs
- 1/2 tsp sriracha
- 1/2 tsp lemon juice
- 5 tbsp butter
- Salt and pepper
- 2 tbsp parsley, minced
- 25 deveined, peeled, cooked shrimp
- 2 sliced onion
- 1/2 cup red bell pepper, minced
- 2 avocado
- 2 bacon slices

Instructions:

1. Whisk fresh eggs, sriracha, lemon juice, and salt in a small bowl.
2. Place butter in a large pan on medium heat.
3. When it melts, add fresh eggs.
4. Cook until slightly firm, lifting the bottom periodically to prevent sticking.
5. Place the remaining ingredients on top of one half of the omelet.
6. Fold over, and cook until finished. Serve and enjoy.

Black Bean, Cilantro, And Avocado Quesadillas

Ingredients

- Canned black beans with no preservative salt added (One 2 6 -ounce).
- One medium-sized tomato (Dice tomato for use).
- Half of a Jalapeno or Anaheim chili pepper (Dice thinly for use).
- Fresh lemon juice (One tablespoon).
- One medium-sized garlic clove (Mince for use).
- A quarter cup of fresh cilantro (Dice thinly for use).
- Extra virgin olive oil (Two tablespoons).
- 6-inch corn tortillas (Eight).
- A quarter cup of plant-based shredded cheese (Optional).
- One medium-sized avocado (Peel and slice it thinly for use).
- Plant-based sour cream (Optional).

Preparation Method And Steps

1. Mash the black beans using a fork or a potato masher in a mixing bowl.
2. Add one or two tablespoons of the water from cooking the beans. This will make the mixture thick and with lumps.
3. Now put the chili peppers, lemon juice, tomato, garlic, and cilantro to the bowl with the black beans and mash all these together while stirring.
4. Put one teaspoon of olive in a big skillet and begin heating it.
5. Place a half cup of the black beans mixture on two tortillas and spread it evenly.
6. Put the tortillas in the skillet with the beans-covered side looking up.
7. **If you want to, one tablespoon of cheese can be sprinkled on the tortillas before you top that off with an extra tortilla.**
8. Cook these quesadillas for approximately 5 minutes in medium heat. Your goal is to cook till the bottom side turns brown.

9. Turn over carefully and cook the other side for about 5 minutes, until browned.
10. Then remove the quesadilla from the skillet and use some avocado slices to garnish it up, while also adding plant-based sour cream if you want to.
11. Do this process over and over again until you make four quesadillas.

Tuna Quinoa Cakes

Ingredients

- Half cup of mashed sweet potatoes
- Two cans of drained tuna
- A quarter cup of cooked quinoa
- A quarter cup of green onion (chop it up for use).
- Two garlic cloves (Mince for use).
- Lemon juice (One tablespoon)
- One fresh freshfresh eggs
- One-quarter cup of plain yogurt
- Mustard (One tablespoon)

- Cayenne pepper (Half tablespoon)
- Paprika (One tablespoon)
- A half-cup of breadcrumbs

Preparation Method And Steps

1. Mix the tuna with sweet potato in a small bowl.
2. Mix the rest of the ingredients in well and stir.
3. Use your hands to make six cakes.
4. Put these cakes on a baking sheet that has been greased. Then place them in the oven to be baked at 400 degrees for approximately 25 min. in the process of the baking, you should have flipped the cakes over once.

Slow Cooker Seafood Ramen

Ingredients

- 65 oz of seafood/vegetable/chicken broth.
- Approximately 6 oz of ramen
- 2 lb of seafood
- Two green onions (Slice for use).
- Low-sodium soy sauce (Two tablespoons)
- Rice vinegar (Two tablespoons)
- Two garlic cloves (Mince for use).
- A quarter cup of chopped up kale
- Half lb. of sliced tomatoes (Slice for use).
- Sesame oil (Half tablespoon)
- Salt (One tablespoon)
- Pepper (A quarter tablespoon)
- Red pepper flakes (A quarter tablespoon)

Preparation Method And Steps

1. Put all the ingredients in the slow cooker excluding the kale, seafood, and ramen.
2. Stir these ingredients together in order to mix it up well.
3. Cook these on a high gas-level for approximately 5 hours. Or put the gas on low, to cook for approximately 6 hours.
4. At this point add the kale, seafood, and ramen to the mixture now.
5. Then cook all of it for 2 6 -5 0 more minutes.

Slow Grilled Chinese Char Siu Chicken

Ingredients

- A quarter c. of organic brown sugar
- A quarter c. raw honey
- A quarter c. organic ketchup
- A quarter c. gluten-free soy sauce
- Beet powder (Three tablespoons)
- Rice vinegar (Two tablespoons)
- Hoisin sauce, gluten-free (One tablespoon)

- Chinese five-spice powder (A half tablespoon)
- For taste, sea salt.
- For taste, black pepper (Ground it up finely for use).
- Two half lbs. chicken thighs (They should be boneless and skinless).
- Cooking oil

Preparation Method And Steps

1. Mix honey, brown sugar, ketchup, beet powder, soy sauce, vinegar, salt, hoisin sauce, five-spice powder, and pepper well in a mixing bowl.
2. Add chicken to the mixture and toss it together well.
3. Marinate this mixture by covering this up and refrigerating for two days.
4. Grill the chicken with heat until the chicken is completely cooked. To achieve this, cook both sides for about 25 minutes.

Thai Salad Bowls

Ingredients

- Green curry paste (One tablespoon).
- A quarter cup of natural peanut butter
- Freshly chopped ginger (Half tablespoon)
- Honey (Two tablespoons)
- Two chopped-up garlic cloves
- A quarter cup of lightly-packaged cilantro
- Fresh lime juice (Two tablespoons)
- Olive oil (Two tablespoons)
- Water (Two tablespoons)
- To taste, Kosher salt

For the salad –

- Four cups of washed and chopped-up lettuces (Use romaine lettuces or hearty baby lettuces).
- Two cups of washed cabbage (Shred for use).
- One red bell pepper (Wash and thinly slice it for use).

- Four green onions (Wash and thinly slice the green and white parts only for use).
- One cup of cilantro leaves that are packed loosely
- Two cups of washed carrots (Shred for use).
- Two cups of cooked quinoa
- A quarter cup of roughly chopped-up peanuts

Preparation Method And Steps

For the salad dressing –

1. Put all the ingredients together in a blender, or you can alternatively use a food processor.
2. After you do that, puree the mixture until it is quite smooth. (You can also whisk and mix the ingredients in a bowl in order to achieve the same results).

For the salad –

3. In the bottom part of a large mixing bowl, put the lettuce.

4. Then add the rest of the ingredients along with the salad dressing.

5. Toss this in order to coat. (You can also serve the salad in a large bowl with the dressing served on the side).

New Orleans Barbecue Shrimp

Required Ingredients

- Two pounds of raw shrimp (Peel for use)
- A quarter cup of olive oil
- Chopped-up rosemary (One tablespoon)
- Black pepper (One tablespoon)
- Cajun seasoning (Two tablespoons)
- Two garlic cloves (Mince for use).
- Low-sodium Worcestershire sauce (Two tablespoons)
- Hot sauce (Two tablespoons)
- Lemon juice (Two tablespoons)
- One cup of low-sodium beef broth

Preparation Method And Steps

1. Pour olive oil in a big skillet over medium gas heat.
2. Put the rosemary, pepper, garlic, and Cajun seasoning in the skillet. Cook this for approximately two minutes.

3. Add the Worcestershire sauce, lemon juice, shrimp, and hot sauce now, then cook till it is pink.
4. Put the beef broth now and cook for three more minutes.
5. Turn the fire down, take it down from the fire and serve.

Creamy Kabocha Squash And Roasted Red Pepper Pasta

Required Ingredients

- Half c. of raw cashews
- One small kabocha squash
- One garlic head
- A quarter cauliflower (Cut it into large floral patterns).
- Half of a medium-sized onion (Chop it up roughly for use).
- One stalk celery (Chop it up roughly for use).
- One medium-sized carrot (Chop it up roughly for use).
- A quarter c. of drained roasted red peppers
- Nutritional yeast (Two tablespoons)
- You can add a pinch of red pepper flakes, but this is optional.
- Approximately 5 c. of vegetable broth
- To taste, Salt
- To taste, black pepper

- Approximately half of the unpacked fresh basil (Slice for use).
- Two lb. of spaghetti noodles (gluten-free)

Serve with –

- Vegan Parmesan cheese (Optional)
- Fresh basil (Slice for use).
- Black pepper

Preparation Method And Steps

1. The cashews should be soaked in water overnight.
2. The oven should be preheated to 400°F. Then position the rack with the cashews in the oven's middle.
3. Put parchment paper or a silicone mat to line the baking sheet
4. Wash the kabocha squash and dry it.
5. Place it on the baking sheet and then place it in the oven to bake for about 25 minutes.
6. The pan should then be removed from the oven. Then allow the kabocha squash to cool

until you can handle it without burning yourself. (Cut the protruding stems off if there are any).
7. Vertically slice the squash in half.
8. After that, take out the seeds and fiber with a spoon or fork.
9. Now slice up the squash in uniform 2 -inch wedges so that they can cook evenly.
10. Put six or seven squash slices on the baking sheet.
11. Remove the loose skin on the garlic's head with your hands.
12. Now use a sharp knife to cut off a quarter-inch from the top of the garlic. The goal is to expose the cloves' tops.
13. Now put the garlic's head with the cut part facing down on the baking sheet.
14. Add the onions, celery, carrots, and cauliflower florets.
15. Sprinkle a bit of salt and pepper for taste on it.

16. Put back in the oven and about 40 minutes, then flip and mix all of it once or twice during the baking.
17. Make the pasta right before the vegetables are finished cooking.
18. Let the vegetables cool after you have baked them.
19. Now then remove the skin of the kabocha and put it in a high-speed blender.
20. Make use of your hands to squeeze the garlic cloves out of the head and place it in the blender. Also, put the drained cashews which you must have drained before and also put the vegetables that remain on the baking sheet.
21. Also, put the nutritional yeast, pepper, red pepper flakes, two cups of vegetable broth, and roasted red peppers at this moment.

22. Blend this mixture until it is completely smooth. (While doing so, you should also make the sauce less thick)
23. At this point, you should taste the meal and see if you should balance out the seasonings.
24. Now put in the sliced basil.
25. Pulse the basil until it is mixed well with the rest. (Make sure you don't blend this unless the sauce's color will become weird).
26. The pasta should now be drained and added back into the pot.
27. Now pour the pasta over the sauce and mix it up until it combines well.
28. When serving this meal, sprinkle it with basil, fresh Parmesan, and black pepper.

Loaded Cauliflower

Required Ingredients

- 3 lb. cauliflower head (Cut this up in floral patterns)
- Six green onions (Chop it up using only the green and white parts for use).
- Butter (Two tablespoons)
- Three garlic cloves (Mince for use).
- Two oz. of cream cheese
- Sea salt (Half tablespoon)
- Black pepper (Quarter tablespoon)
- Ranch seasoning (One and a half tablespoon).
- A quarter c. of organic heavy whipping cream
- Two c. of grated cheddar cheese
- Four slices sugar-free bacon, (Crumble it for use).
- Olive oil

Preparation Method And Steps

1. Let the oven be preheated to about 426 degrees.
2. Use two tablespoons of olive oil to toss the cauliflower. After that, add the cauliflower to a lined baking sheet.
3. The cauliflower should then be roasted on a baking sheet for approximately 26 minutes. The goal is to make the cauliflower tender and make some parts of it brown.

For the cheese sauce (To be made while the cauliflower is roasting)

4. Put the white parts of the green onions, butter, and garlic cloves in a skillet and cook it on medium heat.
5. This mixture should be sauteed till the onions become translucent (This should be about three minutes).
6. Now add cream cheese, heavy cream, salt, pepper, and ranch seasoning (optional) to the skillet along with the onions, butter, and garlic that's already there.

7. The heat should be turned down to medium-low while the cream cheese melts.
8. To finish the cheese sauce, put in one and a half cups of cheddar cheese and stir.
9. Combine the roasted cauliflower with the cheese sauce and then place that mixture into a baking dish.
10. Use the rest of the cheddar cheese to top this mixture and then roast the cauliflower for about 25 more minutes till it gets soft and tender.
11. For toppings, you can add some of the green parts of the green onions, dollops of sour cream, and the crumbled bacon.

Sweet And Hearty Beef Stew

Required Ingredients

- Eight ounces of pre-sliced mushrooms
- Two pounds of lean stew meat (It should be trimmed of all fat).
- One 2 6-ounce bag of baby carrots
- One 8-ounce can of tomato sauce
- A quarter cup of pure maple syrup
- Cider vinegar (Two Tablespoons)
- Kosher salt (Half Teaspoon)
- Cornstarch (Three Teaspoons)
- Cold water (Three Teaspoons)
- One cup of frozen petite peas (Let it thaw out for use).

Preparation Method And Steps

1. The mushrooms should be placed at the bottom of a slow cooker with about 6 quarts.
2. Place the stew meat and carrots on the mushrooms.

3. Now, combine the maple syrup, vinegar, tomato sauce, and salt in a mixing bowl before pouring this mixture over the meat and vegetables.
4. Cover this and continue to cook on the low heat until the meat and carrots become soft and tender. This will take about 8 hours.
5. Mix the cornstarch and water till you get balance.
6. Finally, stir the cornstarch mixture gently with the peas in the slow cooker until the mixture becomes thicker and the peas heat through. It should take about 6 minutes.

Chocolate Chip Protein Bars

Required Ingredients

- A half-cup of honey
- A half-cup of nut butter (You can use peanut butter or almond butter)
- A half-cup of almond milk
- A quarter cup of chocolate protein powder
- Canola oil (One Tablespoon)
- Pure vanilla extract (One Teaspoon)
- One cup of rolled oats
- Two cups of crisp brown rice cereal
- A half-cup of sliced almonds
- A half-cup of dissected mini chocolate chips.
- Kosher salt (Half Teaspoon)
- Nonstick cooking spray

Preparation Method And Steps

1. A baking dish of 10 -by-10 -inches should be coated with cooking spray and kept aside for a while.
2. The oven should be preheated to about 5 6 0 degrees F.
3. Mix honey, protein powder, canola oil, vanilla, nut butter, and almond milk together in a mixing bowl and put it into the oven.
4. This mixture should be stirred and cooked until it starts to bubble. This should take approximately three minutes.
5. After this, remove it from the fire and keep it aside.
6. Mix the quarter cup of chocolate chips, oats, rice, and salt in a large mixing bowl and toss it well to make sure that the mixture is even.
7. A warm honey mix should then be poured over this mixture while it is stirred gently with a spoon or spatula for a good combination of ingredients.

8. Now place this mixture in a baking dish, cover it with some parchment paper.
9. Then press it into the dish firmly and bake for about 30 minutes.
10. Then sprinkle the rest of the chocolate chips on it and allow it to cool totally.
11. Cut this up into any shape you desire like bars or squares.
12. Serve

Easy Creamy Cajun Shrimp Pasta

Required Ingredients

- Eight oz of linguine pasta
- Olive oil (Two Tablespoons).
- 2 lb. of raw shrimp (The veins should be removed from the shrimp and the shells should also be removed).
- Cajun seasoning or Creole seasoning (One Tablespoon)
- 5 oz of andouille sausage (Slice into 2-inch pieces for use)
- Half c. of chopped red peppers
- Half c. of chopped green peppers
- Half c. of chopped onions (Use yellow or white onions)
- 2 c. of fire-roasted diced tomatoes
- Butter (One Tablespoon)
- Half c. of heavy whipped cream
- Half c. of unsweetened almond milk
- Four oz. of cream cheese (These should be cut up in chunks).

- Half c. of shredded Parmesan Reggiano Cheese

Preparation

First cook your pasta the way you normally would.

1. Now put your shrimp in a mixing bowl along with half a tablespoon of Cajun or Creole seasoning. You have to mix these up well enough in order for the shrimp to be completely coated.
2. The skillet or pan to be used should be put on medium-high heat.
4. Add one teaspoon of olive oil to the skillet.
5. Once the olive oil becomes hot enough, add the shrimp to the pan and cook this for about three minutes on each of its sides till you get a bright pink color. After then put the shrimp aside after you remove it from the pan or skillet.
6. Add another teaspoon of olive oil into the pan.

7. Now put in the green peppers, red peppers, onions, and chopped sausage.
8. Sauté this for about four minutes till the vegetables become soft and tender and the onions are lustrous.
9. The vegetables should then be removed from the skillet and put aside.
10. The heat on the skillet should now be reduced to medium-high. Then butter should be added to the pan till it melts.
11. The heavy cream, cream cheese, Parmesan Reggiano cheese, almond milk, and the rest of the Cajun or Creole seasoning (about half a teaspoon) should now be added to the pan.
12. The sauce should be stirred continuously until the cheese has melted completely. It may be a while though.

13. The fire-roasted tomatoes should now be added into the mix and stirred.
14. Then allow this particular mixture to cool for approximately two minutes.
15. The sausage, shrimp, pasta, and vegetables should be put into the pan now and also whisked and stirred.
16. Cook the pasta for about 6 minutes until it sits well with the mixture.
17. Serve.

Gluten-Free Breakfast Skillet

For the skillet –

- Canola oil (One Tablespoon)
- Half a pound of lean ground beef
- One large russet potato
- A quarter cup of chopped-up purple onion
- Garlic powder (One Teaspoon)
- Smoked paprika (One Teaspoon)
- Jalapeno powder (One Teaspoon)
- Basil (One Teaspoon)
- Black pepper (Half Teaspoon)

For the gravy –

- 30 oz can of pinto beans (Drain this for use).
- A quarter cup of chopped-up tomatoes
- Garlic powder (Half Teaspoon)
- Smoked paprika (Quarter Teaspoon)
- Smoked sea salt (Half Teaspoon)
- A quarter cup of maple syrup

Preparation Method And Steps

1. The oven should be preheated to about 400*F.

2. Mix the grounded up beef with a quarter cup of water and spice in a nonstick pan.
3. The beef should be heated over in the oven till it becomes brown.
4. After that, take it down from the heat.
5. Chop the potatoes and onions while the beef is still cooking up.
6. Mix the chopped up potatoes and onion with the beef mixture in the skillet
7. Put one tablespoon of olive oil in the skillet along with the beef mixture.
8. Now put the mixture into the oven and cook it up for about 5 0 minutes.
9. Prepare some gravy making use of a blender while this is still cooking up over the skillet.
10. Add some pinto beans, tomatoes, spices, and syrup to the gravy and puree it till it's smooth enough.
11. Once 5 0 minutes is up, take this out of the oven and top it with some gravy.

12. Put it back into the oven and take the heat down to 490 degrees F for about 25 more minutes.
13. Take it out of the oven and put some sliced tomatoes with cilantro over it as toppings.
14. Use some cornbread or corn tortillas to enjoy this meal.

Healthy Chicken Taco Soup

Required Ingredients

- Avocado or coconut oil (Half Tablespoon)
- One small yellow onion (Dice to use)
- One small red bell pepper (Dice to use)
- One small green bell pepper (Dice to use)
- 6 cloves of minced garlic
- 2 lb. of chicken breast (The skin and bones should be removed)
- Salt (One and Half Teaspoon)
- Dried oregano (One teaspoon)
- Chipotle powder (One Teaspoon)
- Paprika (One Teaspoon)
- Cumin (Two Teaspoons)
- Black pepper (Quarter Teaspoon)
- 2 – 30 oz can of fire-roasted tomatoes (Dice to use)
- 2 – 4.6 oz cans of green chilies
- Quarter c. of fresh lime juice
- 5 2 oz. of chicken broth

- Cilantro

- Diced red onion
- Lime wedges

Preparation Method And Steps

1. Put a big pot over medium-high heat. And once it is hot enough, put in some coconut oil or you can alternatively use avocado oil.
2. Add the peppers, garlic, and onion to the pot and saute it for about 5 minutes till the onions become translucent.
3. The chicken breast, canned green chilies, canned tomatoes, lime juice, spices, and chicken broth should now be added to the pot and stirred till it is well mixed.
4. The soup should be allowed to be at a rolling boil at the moment. You should reduce the heat to a simmer.
5. Let the soup simmer till the chicken is tender and soft enough to shred easily.
6. Now remove the chicken breast from the soup and place it in a bowl.
7. Shred the meat.

8. Put the shredded chicken back into the soup and stir it up till it is mixed well.
9. Serve it up with some diced red onions, lime wedges, and cilantro.

Citrus Baked Salmon

Required Ingredients

- Four (5 ounces) wild salmon fillets (They should be skinless)
- Olive oil (One tablespoon)
- To taste, add some sea salt
- To taste, add some lemon pepper
- Extract juice from one lemon
- 5 slices of fresh lemon
- 5 slices of fresh orange
- 5 sheets of aluminum foil

Preparation Method And Steps

1. The oven should be preheated to about 5 6 0 degrees.
2. Both sides of the salmon should now be coated with olive oil.
3. Now season the salmon with some sea salt and lemon pepper.
4. The salmon fillets should now be placed into the middle of the aluminum foils.

5. Squeeze or pour some lemon juice over each of the salmon fillets.
6. Each of the salmon fillets should now be covered with an orange slice and also a lemon slice.
7. The sides of the aluminum foil should now be folded over the fish so that the package is completely covered. Then place the package into a baking pan.

8. Repeat the above procedure till all of the salmon has been wrapped up and in the baking sheets.
9. Bake all of this in the oven you should have already preheated for about 5 0 minutes.
    10.   **Serve hot**

Caribbean Steamed Fish

Required Ingredients

- Two lbs. of porgy fish (You can use snapper. It should be thoroughly cleaned up and the scales removed.)
- Extract juice from one lime
- Black pepper (Half Teaspoon)
- Salt (One Teaspoon)
- Three garlic cloves (Two of these cloves should be sliced while the remaining one crushed)
- 30 sprigs of thyme
- Butter (Half Tablespoon)
- Oil (Half Tablespoon)
- Two carrots (These should be sliced thinly for use)
- One red pepper (These should be sliced thinly for use)
- One green pepper (These should be sliced thinly for use)
- One onion (These should be sliced thinly for use)

- 25 okra (Cut off the ends)
- One hot pepper (You can use either habanero, scotch bonnet, etc. Make sure you remove the seeds)
- One and a half cups of water

Preparation Method And Steps

1. The fish should be seasoned with crushed garlic, black pepper, salt, some thyme, and lime juice. Set it aside once it is done.
2. Add some butter and oil to a big bottom pot sitting over medium heat.
3. Wait for the butter to melt and once it does, saute some carrots, onions, and red and green pepper till it becomes soft. It should take approximately 6 minutes.
4. Add some of the garlic slices and peppers again.
5. Cook this for a minute more, or maybe two depending on the state of the meal.
6. Bring the meal to a boil by adding some water.
7. Place the fish onto the pot and put some amounts of vegetables on it.

8. Now put some of the okra and the remaining thyme.
9. Lower the heat a bit and cover the pot up to allow the fish to simmer till it's completely done all over.
10. Take the fish off the heat and serve hot.

Orange And Green Smoothie

Required Ingredients

- One navel orange (It should be peeled and cut up into small quarters)
- One frozen banana
- Two cups of chopped-up kale (The rough stems of the kale should be removed)
- One cup of baby spinach leaves
- Half cup of ice
- Half cup of cold water
- Vitamix blender

Preparation Method And Steps

1. The banana should be peeled and added to the blender.
2. Now add the orange, spinach, and kale.
3. The ice should now be poured over the vegetables and fruits along with the water.
4. Start blending this mix at a low speed while you increase it more and more till the entire thing has been mixed and processed smoothly

5. Serve.

Corn Chowder Con Chile Poblano

Required Ingredients

- Vegetable oil (Two Tablespoons)
- One poblano pepper (This should be sliced thinly and all the seeds removed.)
- One medium-sized onion (Slice to use)
- Two garlic cloves. (Chop it roughly to use).
- 6 corn husks
- 5 medium-sized potatoes (They should be cubed)
- Salt (One Teaspoon)

To serve –

- Corn kernels
- Pumpkin seeds
- Chopped cilantro
- Olive oil
- Freshly ground pepper

Preparation Method And Steps

1. Put oil and sliced poblano chili in a big pot. Leave this on the pot till it begins to become soft.

2. Put some onions and garlic on this and leave to cook to about 6 minutes more.
3. Now add the corn kernels, salt, potatoes, and immerse it in water. Cover it up and allow it to cook for approximately 30 minutes.
4. Use a ladle to add a quarter of the veggies and liquid included to the blender. Then blend this mix until it becomes a liquid completely.
5. Now put some more water in the pot with the remaining vegetables.
6. Taste to see whether you need to adjust the seasoning.
7. Serve this meal with a dash of olive oil, some corn kernels, sprouts, pumpkin seeds, and chopped cilantro.
8. Complete this by sprinkling some sea salt and pepper.

Crispy Potato Tacos

Required Ingredients

- 25 corn tortillas

- One c. of mashed potatoes
- Vegetable oil (Four Tablespoons). You can also make use of avocado oil
- 5 long wooden skewers
  To serve –

- Romaine lettuce/Green cabbage (These should be sliced thinly for use)
- Radishes (These should be sliced thinly for use)

- Cilantro

- Guacamole
- Salsa verde

Preparation Method And Steps

1. To make the tortillas supple, they should be heated over the skillet for approximately 30 seconds of high heat.
2. Whip one spoonful of mashed potatoes in the middle of the tortillas. Then roll the tortillas up and put it up on the long skewer.
3. Repeat this process until you have placed at least three more tacos on the skewer. Do this with all the tortillas.
4. Put one tablespoon of oil in a frying pan over high heat.
5. Once the oil heats up, put like four tacos on it and leave it there to fry until they turn golden brown. Once it is of the right color, turn them over to the other side.
6. Remove the tacos from the fire and place them on a dish lined with a paper towel in order to take away all the extra oil.
7. Do this until all of the tacos are completely done.

8. Put the tacos on a plate and put the toppings on it to serve. They should be crispy by now.

Kale And Broccoli Salmon Burgers

Required Ingredients

- One (30 oz) can of wild salmon (Drain to use)
- Half cup of almond meal
- Two freshfresh eggs
- Lemon juice (Two tablespoons)
- Salt (Half teaspoon)
- Garlic powder (Half teaspoon)

- Pepper
- One and a half cups of kale (Remove the stems and chop it up nicely to use)
- A quarter cup of broccoli florets (Chop it up nicely to use)
- Half cup of chopped onion

- Half cup of parsley (It is not compulsory but if you do use it, make sure you chop it nicely)

Preparation Method And Steps

1. Put the salmon in a bowl
2. Now add thefresh eggs , lemon juice, salt, pepper, and almond meal to the salmon. Stir it well enough to mix well.
3. Put the chopped-up vegetables to this and mix well.
4. Make five patties that are packed tightly from this and put in on a plate which should be lined with aluminum foil.
5. Refrigerate this for 5 0 minutes at least.
6. Heat up a big skillet with oil glazed on it while the patties are being refrigerated.
7. Once the skillet is hot enough, add the burgers and cook this for about 8 minutes on each side till it is brown all over.

Grilled Bulgogi Rice Bowls

Required Ingredients

- Two lbs. of bulgogi beef
- Six minced garlic cloves
- Grated ginger (One teaspoon)
- Half cup of soy sauce
- Honey (Two tablespoons)
- Sesame oil (One tablespoon)
- Mirin (One tablespoon)
- Black pepper (Quarter teaspoon)

For the rice –

- Three and a half cups of water
- Two cups of jasmine rice
- Sesame oil (Two tablespoons)
- Salt (One tablespoon)

For the fixings –

- Iceberg lettuce leaves
- One cup of julienned carrots
- One stalk of green onions (Slice to use)
- One onion (Slice or dice it up to use)
- One stalk of diced bok choy, diced
- Sesame oil (One teaspoon)

Preparation Method And Steps

1. Mix the ginger, garlic, honey, mirin, soy sauce, honey, oil, and pepper in a bowl.
2. Put the meat in a baking dish. You should then sort through the thin slices of meat and cut away any excess fat.
3. Marinade the meat and use your hands to massage it.
4. Now cover this up and place it in the fridge for an hour approximately.
5. Use the time the meat is marinating to prepare your vegetables.

Once the meat has marinated for at least 5 0 minutes, you should start making the rice –

6. Boil three and a half cups of water with two tablespoons of sesame oil, and salt. Once the water has started to boil, add two cups of rice, stir this, and then cover the pot up.

7. Reduce the heat to a moderate level for the rice to cook well enough. After 5 0 minutes, remove the rice from the heat for serving.
8. As the rice is cooking, you should then place the onions, sesame oil, and bok choy in a pan to be stir-fried until the onions are cooked. After that, set this aside.
9. You must have preheated the grill by now. If so, put the bulgogi meat on the grill and put it on medium-high heat.
10. Cook this for about 5 minutes per side until you get a firm texture from the meat.
11. Now put the rice, carrots, bok choy/onion mixture, lettuce, and cooked meat on the table.
12. Now you should make use of the lettuce as a kind of taco to hold your meat and other fixings.

Black Garlic, Sesame, And Shitake Cod

Required Ingredients

- Two frozen Alaskan Cod filet
- One black garlic clove
- Olive oil (Two tablespoons)
- Sesame seeds (One teaspoon)
- Half c. of dried shiitake (Re-hydrate and/or water this for use)

Preparation Method And Steps

1. You should preheat the oven to about 46 0F.
2. Now rinse the grime and blood that may be on the frozen fish, and place it on a non-stick pan after drying it off.
3. Put the black garlic clove in a bowl and warm it in the microwave for about 25 seconds.
4. The garlic clove should now be mashed with added olive oil and sesame seeds.
5. This mix should be brushed on the frozen fillets. Then sprinkle some mushrooms on the fillets.
6. Put the fish in the oven for about 30 minutes.

7. Once done, serve it with rice, salad, or any healthy main dish you choose.

Healthy Mexican Casserole

Required Ingredients

- One lb. of chicken breasts (These should be chopped up into small mouthfuls for use)
- One cup of uncooked brown rice or quinoa
- Olive oil (Two tablespoons)
- One bell pepper (Dice to use)
- One white onion (Dice to use)

- Half cup of spinach (You can also use kale, these should be chopped up for use)
- Two minced garlic cloves
- One can of black beans
- One can of fire-roasted tomatoes
- One cup of plain nonfat Greek yogurt
- A quarter cup of mozzarella cheese
- Half cup of cheddar cheese
- Chili powder (Two tablespoons)
- Cayenne pepper (Half teaspoon)

- Cumin seeds (One teaspoon)
- Salt (Half teaspoon)
- Black pepper (Half teaspoon)

Preparation Method And Steps

1. The oven should be preheated to about 5 6 0 degrees F.
2. Two tablespoons of olive oil should now be heated in a skillet. The heat should be medium-high.
3. Cook the cut-up chicken breasts in the skillet until the breasts are not pink in the center anymore. This should take about 6 minutes on each side.
4. As the chicken breasts cook, take the opportunity to add the seasonings and the roughages (onions, garlic, and pepper). Cook this for a bit until the onions and peppers before soft and tender enough.
5. Now make the brown rice or quinoa in a large pot by adding two cups of water to a cup of raw rice or quinoa. Make this boil and then lower the heat, allowing the rice or quinoa to simmer. Cover this for about 30 minutes.
6. Mix the chicken, pepper, and onions with the pot of rice or quinoa.

7. The cans of black beans and fire-roasted diced tomatoes should be added to the pot pf spinach and cooked for approximately two minutes.
8. Mix in the Greek yogurt, a quarter cup of cheddar cheese, and a half cup of mozzarella cheese. Stir this mixture well enough till it combines well, then pour this into a casserole dish (The dish should first be sprayed with non-stick cooking spray).
9. The remaining cheese should now be sprinkled on the casserole and baked for about 25 minutes.
10. Take this out of the oven and let it cool off before you serve.

Shrimp Lettuce Wraps

Required Ingredients

- One romaine lettuce hearts
- Quarter c. of low-sodium chicken broth
- Hoisin sauce (One tablespoon)
- Low-sodium soy sauce (One teaspoon)
- Rice vinegar (Half teaspoon)
- Asian sesame oil (Quarter teaspoon)
- Chili garlic sauce (One and a half teaspoon)
- Cornstarch (Half teaspoon)
- Canola oil (One tablespoon)
- A quarter cup of 5 0 grams cashews
- Six oz of shrimp (It should cut up into small cubes and the veins should be removed)
- One large minced garlic clove
- Half large red bell pepper
- Three green onions (Slice to use, only the white and green parts will be required)

- Cilantro
- One shredded carrot

Preparation Method And Steps

1. Split the lettuce into different leaves and keep it to the side.

2. The chicken broth, soy sauce, rice vinegar, chili, garlic sauce, cornstarch, and hoisin sauce should be mixed in a bowl.
3. Half a tablespoon of canola or avocado oil should put over a skillet to heat till it's about to smoke.
4. Now place the shrimp in the skillet and stir-fry it till it becomes brown. This should be about two minutes.
5. Now put the shrimp on a plate and discard excess liquids from the skillet.
6. Heat another half tablespoon of oil over the same skillet.
7. Now add the bell peppers, green onions, carrots, and garlic to the skillets and stir-fry till they are all crisp and tender. This should take about 2 minutes.

8. Put the shrimp back into the pan, and then add the cilantro and also cashews.
9. The soy-sauce mixture should then be added to the pan and also stir-fried till the shrimp is completely well cooked. This should take three minutes.
10. To serve, place the shrimp mixture onto the lettuce leaves.

Shakshuka

Required Ingredients

- Olive oil (Two tablespoons)
- One cup of diced yellow onion
- One jalapeno pepper
- One cup of diced yellow bell pepper
- One cup of diced green zucchini
- One cup of diced yellow summer squash
- Two big garlic cloves (Mince to use)
- Ground cumin (One teaspoon)
- Turmeric (Half teaspoon)
- Sweet paprika (One teaspoon)
- 28 ounces of diced tomatoes
- Tomato paste (Two tablespoons)
- Honey (Two teaspoons)
- Cider vinegar (One teaspoon)
- One cup of corn
- Kosher salt (Half teaspoon)
- Freshly ground pepper
- A quarter cup of crumbled feta cheese
- Four big pasteurized freshfresh eggs
- Chopped parsley (optional)

- Zaatar (Optional)

Preparation Method And Steps

1. Put some olive oil over the skillet and heat it up with medium heat.
2. Put some onions on the skillets and saute it for about two minutes.
3. Put some jalapeno peppers and bell peppers to this and sauté for about four minutes.
4. Add the zucchini and summer squash, then sauté for five minutes.
5. Next up, put the garlic in along with the turmeric, paprika, cumin. Stir this mixture until it is smelling great. It usually just takes a minute.
6. The heat should now be reduced to medium so that you can add the tomatoes, honey, corn, tomato paste, and cider vinegar. Add the salt and pepper in while you stir this.
7. Let this simmer for approximately 25 minutes.

8. Turn off the fire, and press the feta that has been crumbled into the tomato sauce. Use the back of a spoon to make four marks on the sauce.

9. Break four freshfresh eggs one by one and put them consecutively into the four indentations. Then with a spatula, drag through the fresh freshfresh eggs whites without spoiling the yolks.

10. Let this simmer in low heat for approximately five minutes as you continue to baste the freshfresh eggs and gently stir the sauce.
11. Cover this up and cook for about seven minutes more.
12. Serve this meal with parsley and zaatar sprinkled over it.

Coconut Steel-Cut Oatmeal With Almonds And Dark Chocolate

Required Ingredients

- Two cups of rolled oats
- Four cups of unsweetened coconut milk
- Sea salt
- Half cup of unsweetened coconut
- Half cup of chopped almonds
- A quarter cup of chopped dark chocolate
- Honey

Preparation Method And Steps

1. Mix the oats and coconut milk with a pinch of sea salt in a large container with a lid.

2. Keep it in a fridge all night.

3. Once it's morning, you can then enjoy your oats cold or warm it up for a minute or two. You can top it with dark chocolate, coconut, and almonds with some honey for sweetening.

Crunchy Roasted Chickpeas

Required Ingredients

- One can (2 6 -oz) of chickpeas
- Canola oil (One tablespoon)
- Sea salt (One teaspoon)
- Black pepper (One teaspoon)

Preparation Method And Steps

1. The oven should be preheated to about 490 degrees.
2. The chickpeas should then be rinsed and drained. Right after that, dry them off to make it easier for cooking.
3. Mix the chickpeas, salt, pepper, and oil in a bowl and stir it up.
4. The baking sheet should now be coated with cooking spray. After that, put the chickpeas on there and place it in the oven.
5. Bake this for about 5 6 minutes till the chickpeas are crispy.

Crispy Baked Falafel

Required Ingredients

- One c. of dried chickpeas
- Half c. of fresh parsley
- Half chopped medium-sized onion chopped
- Three chopped garlic cloves
- Cumin (One teaspoon)
- Coriander (One teaspoon)
- Black pepper (Quarter teaspoon)
- Salt (One teaspoon)
- Quarter c. of vegetable oil

Preparation Method And Steps

1. The oven should be preheated to about 400F.
2. Drain the chickpeas and rinse them with clean water once they are through soaking.
3. The chickpeas, onions, spices, garlic, parsley, pepper, and salt should then be added to a food processor and pulsed till there's a consistent texture.
4. Use your hands to make about 25 small falafel balls.

5. Put some canola oil on a medium pan and heat it up. (You can also use vegetable oil).

6. Add the falafel balls to this.
7. Fry the falafel balls in the oil till they are completely fried. It should take about two minutes each.
8. After frying, add the balls to the lined baking sheet.
9. The remaining oil on the pan should then be drizzled over the falafel balls before they are baked for like 25 minutes.
10. This can be enjoyed with your best food pairings like greens, rice, etc.

CPSIA information can be obtained
at www.ICGtesting.com
Printed in the USA
LVHW081553120222
710987LV00022B/515

9 781990 061837